UNDERSTANDING BELL'S PALSY

Comprehensive Guide To Causes, Symptoms, Diagnosis, Treatment Options, And Recovery Strategies For Facial Paralysis

DR. LINCOLN WAYLON

DISCLAIMER

This book contains information that should only be used for educational and informational reasons; it is not meant to be used as a source of medical or psychological advice. The author's studies, life experiences, and expertise in the area of health and wellness served as the foundation for the content. It should not, however, be used in place of expert counsel, a diagnosis, or medical care.

Any queries you may have about a physical or mental health issue should always be directed toward the advice of a licensed healthcare provider or mental health specialist. With regard to the efficacy or outcomes of the methods or suggestions included in this book, the author and publisher make no representations or warranties.

Any information or methods in this book are used entirely at the reader's own risk and discretion. The material provided here may be used or misused, and neither the author nor the publisher will be held responsible for any results, losses, or negative impacts.

Keep in mind that everyone has different demands and reactions to health and wellness routines. Any health and wellness plans you implement must be customized to your particular circumstances, and you should speak with experts to make sure the plans meet your needs.

TABLE OF CONTENTS

ABOUT THE BOOK

"Understanding Bell's Palsy" offers a comprehensive and insightful exploration of this complex condition, vital for both patients and healthcare professionals. With a thorough overview, the book delves into the fundamental aspects of Bell's Palsy, defining its medical terminology and tracing the historical evolution of our understanding. It highlights the key symptoms and signs, the profound impact on daily life, and the emotional and psychological dimensions that accompany this condition. This foundation sets the stage for a deeper appreciation of the multifaceted nature of Bell's Palsy and its effects on individuals.

In examining the causes and risk factors, the book provides an in-depth analysis of the roles of viral infections, autoimmune responses, and genetic predispositions. It also considers environmental and lifestyle influences, as well as pre-existing medical conditions that may contribute to the onset of Bell's Palsy. This thorough exploration is essential for understanding the diverse factors that can lead to the development of this condition, offering readers a holistic view of its etiology.

The diagnostic process is a critical component of effective management, and the book covers this in detail. It outlines the initial assessment and symptoms review, the role of various diagnostic tests like MRI and CT scans, and the importance of differentiating Bell's Palsy from other conditions. The involvement of specialists such as neurologists and ENT doctors is emphasized, underscoring the need for a comprehensive evaluation to ensure accurate diagnosis and appropriate treatment.

Treatment and management strategies are thoroughly examined, including standard medication options, the use of corticosteroids and antiviral drugs, and the role of non-pharmacological treatments like physiotherapy.

The book also addresses home care strategies and lifestyle modifications, providing practical advice for managing Bell's Palsy effectively.

This section is designed to equip readers with a range of tools to support their recovery and daily well-being.

Physical therapy and rehabilitation are crucial for many individuals with Bell's Palsy. The book details the goals of physical therapy, the types of exercises and techniques, and the significance of facial muscle exercises. It highlights the importance of collaboration with physical therapists and offers guidance on tracking progress and adjusting therapy as needed, ensuring that readers have a clear understanding of how to optimize their rehabilitation efforts.

Alternative and complementary therapies are explored as well, including popular treatments like acupuncture, herbal remedies, and mind-body techniques such as meditation and yoga. The book evaluates the effectiveness and safety of these approaches, providing a balanced perspective on how they may complement conventional treatments and support overall recovery.

Managing complications is another essential aspect covered in the book. It addresses common complications, strategies for managing facial pain and discomfort, and how to cope with issues related to facial weakness. Emotional and psychological challenges are also discussed, with advice on seeking additional medical support when necessary.

The long-term outlook and prognosis section provides valuable insights into expected recovery rates, potential long-term effects, and factors that influence prognosis. The importance of ongoing medical follow-up is emphasized, alongside the need for support networks and resources to aid in managing the long-term aspects of Bell's Palsy.

Living with Bell's Palsy presents unique challenges, and the book offers practical advice on adjusting to daily life, coping with social and work-related issues, and maintaining mental health and well-being. It also highlights the importance of engaging with patient communities and support groups, offering a comprehensive guide for navigating the complexities of living with this condition.

Addressing common concerns through detailed FAQs, the book answers critical questions such as early signs of Bell's Palsy, differentiation from stroke, effective treatments, the possibility of recurrence, and finding support and resources. This section ensures that readers have access to essential information and guidance for managing their condition effectively.

CHAPTER ONE

OVERVIEW OF BELL'S PALSY

DEFINITION AND MEDICAL TERMINOLOGY

Bell's Palsy is a neurological condition characterized by sudden, temporary weakness or paralysis of the facial muscles, usually affecting one side of the face. This condition occurs due to inflammation of the facial nerve, known as cranial nerve VII, which controls the muscles of facial expression.

The precise cause of the inflammation is often unknown, but it is believed to be related to viral infections, such as those caused by herpes simplex virus. In medical terminology, Bell's Palsy is classified as a form of facial nerve dysfunction that leads to unilateral facial droop, impacting expressions such as smiling or closing the eye on the affected side.

The condition is typically diagnosed through clinical evaluation, where a physician assesses the characteristic symptoms and rules out other potential causes of facial paralysis, such as stroke or tumors. Electromyography (EMG) and imaging studies may be employed to further evaluate nerve function and exclude other conditions. Bell's Palsy is differentiated from other facial nerve disorders by its abrupt onset, absence of other neurological deficits, and the fact that the symptoms often peak within 48 hours.

Treatment often involves corticosteroids to reduce inflammation and swelling of the facial nerve, which can help speed up recovery and improve outcomes. In some cases, physical therapy may be recommended to help patients regain facial muscle strength and coordination. The prognosis is generally favorable, with many individuals experiencing significant improvement or full recovery within three to six months.

HISTORICAL CONTEXT AND EVOLUTION OF KNOWLEDGE

The recognition of Bell's Palsy dates back to the early 19th century, with the condition being named after

Sir Charles Bell, a Scottish surgeon who made significant contributions to the understanding of the facial nerve. In 1821, Bell provided a detailed description of the condition, differentiating it from other types of facial paralysis and establishing the basis for further research. The early understanding of Bell's Palsy was limited, with the condition often being considered idiopathic, meaning the cause was unknown.

Over the decades, advances in medical science have led to a more comprehensive understanding of the condition. The development of neuroimaging techniques and improved diagnostic tools has allowed for better visualization of the facial nerve and identification of potential causes of inflammation. Research into viral infections and their role in Bell's Palsy has provided insights into the mechanisms underlying the condition, leading to more targeted treatments and management strategies.

The historical evolution of knowledge has also led to the development of standardized diagnostic criteria and treatment protocols, improving the consistency of care and outcomes for patients. Ongoing research continues to refine our understanding of Bell's Palsy, with a focus on identifying risk factors, optimizing treatment approaches, and exploring potential long-term effects.

KEY SYMPTOMS AND SIGNS

The primary symptom of Bell's Palsy is a sudden onset of facial weakness or paralysis on one side of the face, which may be accompanied by drooping of the mouth and difficulty closing the eye on the affected side. Patients often experience a sensation of numbness or tingling in the face and may have difficulty with facial expressions such as smiling or frowning. The condition can also affect the ability to taste on the front two-thirds of the tongue and cause increased sensitivity to sound in one ear.

In addition to these core symptoms, Bell's Palsy may present with other signs such as pain or discomfort around the jaw or behind the ear, which often precedes the onset of facial weakness. Some individuals report a feeling of fullness in the affected ear or altered sensation in the face. The rapid progression of symptoms, usually reaching their peak within 48 hours, is a hallmark feature of Bell's Palsy and helps differentiate it from other forms of facial paralysis.

It is important for individuals experiencing these symptoms to seek medical evaluation promptly, as early diagnosis and treatment can improve outcomes. While the majority of patients with Bell's Palsy recover fully or significantly within a few months, early intervention can help mitigate complications and support the rehabilitation process.

IMPACT ON DAILY LIFE

Bell's Palsy can have a profound impact on daily life, affecting both physical and social aspects. The facial weakness or paralysis can make basic activities such as eating, drinking, and speaking challenging, as individuals may have difficulty controlling the affected side of their mouth. This can lead to frustration and a decrease in the quality of life, as tasks that were previously taken for granted become more complex and time-consuming.

Social interactions can also be affected, as changes in facial appearance and expressions may lead to self-consciousness and altered social dynamics. Individuals with Bell's Palsy may feel embarrassed or anxious about their appearance, which can impact their confidence and relationships with others. In some cases, the visible symptoms may lead to misunderstandings or misjudgments from others, further contributing to emotional distress.

The impact of Bell's Palsy extends beyond the immediate physical symptoms, affecting an individual's overall well-being and daily functioning. Support from healthcare professionals, family, and friends can play a crucial role in helping individuals cope with these challenges and adapt to the temporary changes in their lives.

EMOTIONAL AND PSYCHOLOGICAL ASPECTS

The emotional and psychological impact of Bell's Palsy can be significant, with many individuals experiencing a range of feelings from anxiety and frustration to depression.

The sudden onset of facial paralysis and the resulting changes in appearance can lead to a sense of loss of control and uncertainty about the future. These feelings are often compounded by the social implications of the condition, as individuals may struggle with self-esteem and body image issues.

The stress and emotional strain of dealing with Bell's Palsy can affect mental health and overall well-being. Some individuals may experience heightened levels of anxiety or depression due to the condition's impact on their daily lives and social interactions. Individuals need to seek support from mental health professionals if they are struggling with emotional challenges related to Bell's Palsy.

Support groups and counseling can be valuable resources for individuals coping with the psychological aspects of Bell's Palsy. Connecting with others who have experienced similar challenges can provide a sense of community and understanding, helping individuals navigate the emotional and psychological impact of the condition while working towards recovery.

CHAPTER TWO

CAUSES AND RISK FACTORS

VIRAL INFECTIONS AND THEIR ROLE

Viral infections are a primary cause of Bell's Palsy, particularly those affecting the upper respiratory tract. The herpes simplex virus (HSV), which is responsible for cold sores, is commonly implicated in this condition. This virus can become latent in the body and reactivate, leading to inflammation and swelling of the facial nerve. This inflammation disrupts the nerve's function, causing sudden facial weakness or paralysis. It is essential to recognize symptoms of viral infections early, as timely treatment can potentially reduce the risk of developing Bell's Palsy.

Additionally, other viral infections like influenza and Epstein-Barr virus have been linked to Bell's Palsy. These viruses can trigger an immune response that inadvertently affects the facial nerve.

Understanding the connection between these viral infections and Bell's Palsy helps in diagnosing and managing the condition effectively. If a person experiences facial drooping or weakness following a viral illness, medical evaluation is crucial to determine if it is related to Bell's Palsy.

Preventive measures, such as maintaining good hygiene and seeking prompt treatment for viral infections, can reduce the risk of Bell's Palsy. Early intervention with antiviral medications and supportive care may help manage symptoms and potentially minimize nerve damage. Regular check-ups and monitoring for signs of reactivation in individuals with a history of viral infections are recommended to manage and prevent complications associated with Bell's Palsy.

AUTOIMMUNE RESPONSES

Autoimmune responses occur when the body's immune system mistakenly attacks its tissues, including the facial nerve.

In the case of Bell's Palsy, the immune system may target the facial nerve, leading to inflammation and paralysis. This can be triggered by various factors, including infections or stress, which can make the immune system more reactive. Identifying autoimmune conditions as a cause of Bell's Palsy involves thorough medical evaluation to distinguish it from other possible causes.

For individuals with a history of autoimmune diseases, such as rheumatoid arthritis or lupus, the risk of developing Bell's Palsy might be higher. Managing these autoimmune conditions through medication and lifestyle changes can help mitigate the risk. Treatments might include corticosteroids to reduce inflammation and immunosuppressive drugs to control the autoimmune response. Regular consultations with healthcare providers are necessary to adjust treatment plans and monitor the condition effectively.

Understanding the link between autoimmune responses and Bell's Palsy aids in tailoring treatment strategies. For example, immunotherapy or specific autoimmune disease management can be crucial in addressing the underlying cause. Educating patients about managing autoimmune diseases and recognizing early symptoms of Bell's Palsy can improve outcomes and provide a clearer pathway for treatment and recovery.

GENETIC FACTORS AND FAMILY HISTORY

Genetic factors play a significant role in the predisposition to Bell's Palsy. Individuals with a family history of the condition may have a higher risk due to inherited genetic traits. Although specific genes related to Bell's Palsy have not been definitively identified, familial patterns suggest that genetics can influence susceptibility. Family history is a critical component in assessing risk, and patients with close relatives who have experienced Bell's Palsy should discuss this with their healthcare providers.

Genetic predisposition can interact with environmental and viral factors, compounding the risk. Understanding family history helps in early detection and preventive strategies, such as more vigilant monitoring of facial nerve health and proactive management of potential symptoms. Genetic counseling may be beneficial for families with multiple cases of Bell's Palsy, providing insights into hereditary risks and informed decision-making.

While genetic factors are not modifiable, awareness of family history allows for better preparedness and personalized care. Individuals with a genetic predisposition can benefit from early intervention strategies, such as regular check-ups and immediate treatment if symptoms of Bell's Palsy arise. This proactive approach can help in managing the condition more effectively and improving overall outcomes.

ENVIRONMENTAL AND LIFESTYLE FACTORS

Environmental and lifestyle factors also contribute to the risk of Bell's Palsy. Stress, exposure to cold temperatures, and physical trauma are among the environmental factors that may trigger or exacerbate the condition. High stress levels can weaken the immune system, making the body more susceptible to infections and inflammation that can affect the facial nerve. Lifestyle choices, such as smoking and excessive alcohol consumption, can further increase risk.

Taking steps to manage stress and maintain a healthy lifestyle can help reduce the risk of Bell's Palsy. Implementing stress-reducing techniques, such as meditation and exercise, alongside avoiding extreme cold exposure, can be beneficial. Additionally, adopting a balanced diet and avoiding harmful substances contribute to overall health and potentially lower the risk of developing Bell's Palsy.

Monitoring environmental exposures and making lifestyle adjustments can have a significant impact on reducing Bell's Palsy risk. For those already affected, addressing lifestyle factors and managing stress can support recovery and improve outcomes. Regular health check-ups and lifestyle modifications should be considered as part of a comprehensive approach to preventing and managing Bell's Palsy.

PRE-EXISTING MEDICAL CONDITIONS

Pre-existing medical conditions can influence the likelihood of developing Bell's Palsy. Conditions such as diabetes, which affects nerve health, and hypertension, which may contribute to inflammation, can increase susceptibility to facial nerve issues. Managing these conditions effectively is crucial in reducing the risk of complications such as Bell's Palsy. Regular monitoring and treatment of underlying health issues are important for overall nerve health.

For individuals with chronic health conditions, maintaining good control over their medical status is essential. This might involve adhering to prescribed treatments, lifestyle modifications, and routine medical evaluations. Proper management of pre-existing conditions can prevent complications that might contribute to the onset of Bell's Palsy.

Incorporating strategies to manage pre-existing medical conditions can enhance overall health and reduce the risk of developing Bell's Palsy. Collaborative care with healthcare providers to address these conditions proactively supports better outcomes and reduces the likelihood of complications affecting facial nerve function.

CHAPTER THREE

DIAGNOSIS

INITIAL ASSESSMENT AND SYMPTOMS REVIEW

The initial assessment for Bell's Palsy involves a thorough review of symptoms and a detailed patient history. This typically begins with the patient describing the onset and progression of their facial weakness, which usually appears suddenly on one side of the face.

Common symptoms include drooping of the mouth, inability to close the eye on the affected side, and changes in facial expressions. It's crucial to note if there are associated symptoms like pain around the jaw or behind the ear, which can help differentiate Bell's Palsy from other conditions.

A comprehensive symptom review also considers the patient's medical history and recent events. For instance, recent infections, such as upper respiratory or viral infections, may be relevant as they could be linked to the development of Bell's Palsy. Additionally, the presence of any prior neurological issues or similar episodes can provide context. The information gathered helps in establishing a baseline for further diagnostic evaluation and tailoring the treatment approach.

During the assessment, physical examination focuses on facial movements. The clinician evaluates the symmetry of the face by asking the patient to perform various facial expressions, such as raising their eyebrows, smiling, and closing their eyes tightly. This examination helps identify the extent of facial muscle weakness and whether it is consistent with Bell's Palsy or if further investigation is required.

DIAGNOSTIC TESTS (E.G., MRI, CT SCANS)

Diagnostic tests are essential in confirming Bell's Palsy and ruling out other potential causes of facial paralysis. Magnetic Resonance Imaging (MRI) is often used to visualize the facial nerve and surrounding structures.

MRI can help identify any abnormalities or lesions on the facial nerve that could be causing the symptoms. It provides detailed images of the brain and nerve pathways, which is crucial for accurate diagnosis.

Computed Tomography (CT) scans are another diagnostic tool used to examine the bony structures around the facial nerve. Although CT scans are less detailed than MRI in soft tissue imaging, they can detect any structural abnormalities, such as fractures or tumors, that might affect the facial nerve. CT scans are particularly useful in emergencies or when MRI is not available.

In addition to these imaging tests, electromyography (EMG) may be employed to assess the electrical activity of facial muscles. This test can help determine the severity of nerve damage and guide treatment options. Combining these diagnostic tools ensures a comprehensive evaluation and helps rule out other conditions that may present with similar symptoms.

Differential diagnosis is crucial to exclude other conditions that may present with facial paralysis. Conditions such as stroke, tumors, or infections need to be considered, as they can have similar initial presentations.

A stroke, for example, often affects both the upper and lower parts of the face on one side and is usually accompanied by other neurological symptoms like speech difficulties or weakness in other body parts.

Other conditions to rule out include Lyme disease, which can cause facial paralysis but is often accompanied by other symptoms like a rash or a history of tick bites. Ramsay Hunt syndrome, another condition associated with facial paralysis, is caused by the varicella-zoster virus and may present with a painful rash in the ear or mouth. Accurate differential diagnosis involves comparing the patient's symptoms with the characteristics of these conditions and using diagnostic tests to confirm or exclude them.

The process involves careful analysis of patient history, symptom presentation, and results from diagnostic tests. The goal is to ensure that the facial paralysis is indeed due to Bell's Palsy and not another condition requiring different management or treatment strategies. This thorough approach minimizes the risk of misdiagnosis and ensures appropriate care.

ROLE OF SPECIALISTS (NEUROLOGISTS, ENT DOCTORS)

Specialists play a vital role in the diagnosis and management of Bell's Palsy. Neurologists are often the primary specialists involved, as they have expertise in disorders affecting the nervous system. They perform detailed neurological evaluations to assess the extent of facial nerve involvement and determine the most appropriate treatment plan. Their expertise is crucial in differentiating Bell's Palsy from other neurological conditions and managing any complications.

Otolaryngologists, or ENT doctors, also contribute significantly, particularly in cases where the facial paralysis might be related to issues in the ear or throat. They evaluate the patient for any infections or abnormalities in the ear that could be contributing to the facial symptoms. ENT specialists are also involved in managing any associated symptoms, such as difficulty with taste or salivation, which may be part of Bell's Palsy presentation.

In complex or severe cases, a multidisciplinary approach involving both neurologists and ENT specialists ensures comprehensive care.

This collaboration helps in devising a treatment plan that addresses all aspects of the condition and supports optimal recovery. The combined expertise of these specialists provides a thorough evaluation and targeted treatment for Bell's Palsy.

IMPORTANCE OF A COMPREHENSIVE EVALUATION

A comprehensive evaluation is essential in the management of Bell's Palsy to ensure an accurate diagnosis and effective treatment plan. This thorough assessment includes a detailed patient history, physical examination, and appropriate diagnostic tests. By considering all aspects of the patient's symptoms and medical background, healthcare providers can accurately diagnose Bell's Palsy and rule out other potential causes of facial paralysis.

Comprehensive evaluation also involves monitoring the progression of the condition and response to treatment. Regular follow-ups and assessments help in tracking improvements or detecting any complications early. This ongoing evaluation is crucial for adjusting treatment strategies as needed and ensuring the best possible outcome for the patient.

Furthermore, a detailed evaluation helps in addressing any patient concerns and providing education about the condition. Understanding the nature of Bell's Palsy, potential complications, and expected recovery timelines empowers patients and helps them manage their condition effectively. Overall, a thorough evaluation lays the foundation for effective treatment and supports the patient's journey toward recovery.

CHAPTER FOUR

TREATMENT AND MANAGEMENT

STANDARD MEDICATION OPTIONS

When addressing Bell's Palsy, corticosteroids are commonly prescribed to reduce inflammation and improve recovery. Prednisone is the most frequently used corticosteroid for this condition. It helps to alleviate the swelling of the facial nerve, which can relieve symptoms such as facial weakness and discomfort. Typically, a high dose is administered initially, followed by a tapering dose over a few weeks. This treatment is usually most effective when started within the first 72 hours of symptom onset.

Antiviral medications are sometimes considered, especially if a viral infection, such as herpes simplex, is suspected to contribute to Bell's Palsy. Acyclovir or valacyclovir may be used in combination with corticosteroids to combat the viral cause. However, the benefit of antiviral drugs in the treatment of Bell's Palsy is still debated, and they are not universally prescribed for all patients. The decision to use antivirals depends on clinical judgment and the presence of viral symptoms.

In addition to corticosteroids and antivirals, pain relievers such as acetaminophen or ibuprofen can help manage discomfort associated with Bell's Palsy. These medications address pain and reduce fever, if present, providing symptomatic relief. They do not affect the underlying condition but can make the patient more comfortable during the recovery period.

CORTICOSTEROIDS AND THEIR EFFECTS

Corticosteroids are essential in managing Bell's Palsy due to their potent anti-inflammatory properties. Prednisone, the most commonly used corticosteroid, works by decreasing the inflammation around the facial nerve. This reduction in inflammation can significantly improve facial muscle function and reduce symptoms of weakness or paralysis. The drug is typically given in a tapered dose over a few weeks, starting with a higher dose and gradually reducing it to minimize side effects.

The effectiveness of corticosteroids is most pronounced when treatment begins early, ideally within the first three days of symptom onset. Studies have shown that patients who receive corticosteroids early in the course of Bell's Palsy have a better chance of a full recovery compared to those who start treatment later. It's important to follow the prescribed dosage and duration to maximize benefits and avoid potential side effects such as weight gain or high blood pressure.

Corticosteroids may also help to alleviate associated symptoms like pain or discomfort around the face. By reducing inflammation, they can minimize nerve irritation, which contributes to overall symptom relief. Patients should be monitored for any adverse reactions, and regular follow-ups with the healthcare provider are necessary to adjust treatment as needed and ensure optimal recovery.

ROLE OF ANTIVIRAL DRUGS

Antiviral drugs can be prescribed if a viral infection, such as herpes simplex, is suspected to be involved in Bell's Palsy. These medications, including acyclovir and valacyclovir, work by inhibiting the replication of the virus, potentially reducing the severity and duration of the symptoms.

The use of antivirals is based on the hypothesis that viral infection plays a role in the development of Bell's Palsy, though their effectiveness varies and remains a topic of debate.

The decision to use antiviral drugs is often made based on clinical judgment and the presence of additional symptoms that suggest a viral cause. In some cases, antivirals are combined with corticosteroids to address both inflammation and viral factors. However, the overall benefit of antivirals in improving outcomes for Bell's Palsy patients is still under review, and they are not universally recommended.

Patients taking antiviral medications should be aware of potential side effects, such as gastrointestinal issues or allergic reactions. It's important to complete the full course of medication as prescribed to ensure the best possible outcome. Regular communication with a healthcare provider helps in monitoring the effectiveness and managing any adverse effects that may arise during treatment.

NON-PHARMACOLOGICAL TREATMENTS (E.G., PHYSIOTHERAPY)

Non-pharmacological treatments, particularly physiotherapy, play a crucial role in the rehabilitation of Bell's Palsy. Physiotherapy focuses on facial exercises that help to strengthen the facial muscles and improve coordination. This can aid in regaining facial symmetry and functionality. Exercises typically include facial movements such as raising eyebrows, closing eyes tightly, and smiling. A physiotherapist can guide patients through a tailored exercise program based on individual needs.

In addition to exercises, techniques like massage and facial heat application can promote circulation and reduce muscle stiffness. These methods help to alleviate pain and discomfort while supporting muscle recovery. Regular physiotherapy sessions are recommended to track progress and adjust the treatment plan as necessary, ensuring that exercises are performed correctly and effectively.

Home-based exercises and physiotherapy routines should be complemented by consistent practice. Patients are encouraged to perform exercises multiple times a day to maximize benefits. Adherence to the prescribed routine is key to achieving optimal recovery and improving facial muscle function over time.

HOME CARE STRATEGIES AND LIFESTYLE MODIFICATIONS

Home care strategies for Bell's Palsy include managing symptoms and making lifestyle adjustments to support recovery.

Facial exercises should be incorporated into daily routines to enhance muscle strength and coordination. Patients may also benefit from using facial moisturizers to prevent dryness and irritation, especially if the ability to blink is impaired.

Lifestyle modifications include maintaining a healthy diet and ensuring adequate rest, which are essential for overall recovery and well-being. Avoiding exposure to extreme temperatures and protecting the face from wind and sun can prevent further irritation. It's also advisable to avoid activities that may strain the facial muscles or exacerbate symptoms.

Regular follow-up with healthcare providers is important to monitor progress and adjust treatment plans as needed. Support from family and friends can also be beneficial, providing encouragement and assisting with daily tasks if needed. By combining medical treatment with effective home care strategies, patients can improve their chances of a full recovery from Bell's Palsy.

CHAPTER FIVE

PHYSICAL THERAPY AND REHABILITATION

GOALS OF PHYSICAL THERAPY

Physical therapy for Bell's Palsy primarily aims to restore normal facial function and symmetry. The primary goal is to improve facial muscle strength and coordination, which can be significantly impacted by the condition.

By engaging in targeted exercises, patients work towards reestablishing the ability to move facial muscles with more precision and ease, reducing the appearance of facial asymmetry and improving overall facial expressions.

Another key objective is to prevent muscle atrophy and maintain muscle tone. Without intervention, affected facial muscles can weaken over time, leading to more pronounced asymmetry and functional difficulties. Through physical therapy, patients can maintain or regain muscle tone, which supports the recovery of normal facial function and minimizes the long-term impact of Bell's Palsy.

Furthermore, physical therapy helps in alleviating discomfort and pain associated with Bell's Palsy. By using techniques that address muscle tension and promote relaxation, physical therapists can reduce the pain and discomfort that often accompanies the condition. This approach not only enhances the quality of life but also facilitates a more effective recovery process.

TYPES OF EXERCISES AND TECHNIQUES

A variety of exercises and techniques are utilized in physical therapy for Bell's Palsy to target different aspects of facial function. These include facial muscle-strengthening exercises, which involve repeated movements designed to increase muscle strength and control. Examples include raising the eyebrows, closing the eyes tightly, and smiling broadly, which help activate and fortify the affected muscles.

Stretching exercises are also integral to the therapy, aimed at improving the flexibility and range of motion of facial muscles. Techniques such as gentle stretching of the facial muscles and massaging the affected areas can reduce stiffness and enhance muscle function. These exercises help to prevent contractures and improve overall facial symmetry.

In addition to strengthening and stretching, facial reeducation techniques are used to retrain the facial muscles and nerves. These techniques involve practicing specific facial movements and expressions to promote neuromuscular coordination and reestablish normal facial expressions. This aspect of therapy is crucial for regaining the ability to perform daily facial expressions and functions effectively.

IMPORTANCE OF FACIAL MUSCLE EXERCISES

Facial muscle exercises play a crucial role in the recovery process for Bell's Palsy by helping to reestablish muscle strength and coordination. These exercises are designed to stimulate the affected muscles, promoting circulation and improving muscle tone. Regularly engaging in these exercises can help counteract muscle weakness and prevent further deterioration of facial function.

Additionally, facial muscle exercises are essential for enhancing facial symmetry and expression. Through consistent practice, patients can work towards achieving a more balanced and symmetrical appearance, which can have a significant impact on self-esteem and social interactions. Improved muscle control also aids in more natural facial expressions and better communication.

The exercises also contribute to overall facial comfort and functionality. By maintaining muscle activity and preventing atrophy, patients can reduce the likelihood of developing contractures or other complications that can arise from prolonged muscle inactivity. This proactive approach supports a smoother recovery and helps in regaining full facial function.

COLLABORATION WITH PHYSICAL THERAPISTS

Working closely with physical therapists is fundamental to achieving optimal outcomes in Bell's Palsy rehabilitation. Physical therapists are trained to design individualized treatment plans that address the specific needs and goals of each patient. They provide expert guidance on the appropriate exercises and techniques to use, ensuring that therapy is tailored to the patient's condition and progress.

Therapists also offer valuable support in monitoring progress and making necessary adjustments to the therapy regimen. They assess the effectiveness of the exercises and techniques, providing feedback and modifications as needed to enhance results. This ongoing evaluation helps to ensure that the therapy remains effective and aligned with the patient's recovery goals.

Furthermore, physical therapists play a crucial role in educating patients about their condition and the importance of adherence to the therapy program.

TRACKING PROGRESS AND ADJUSTING THERAPY

Tracking progress is essential for evaluating the effectiveness of physical therapy and making necessary adjustments. Regular assessments, including measuring facial muscle strength, range of motion, and overall symmetry, help to determine how well the therapy is working. These evaluations guide the physical therapist in identifying areas of improvement and any modifications needed to optimize the treatment plan.

Adjustments to therapy may involve altering the intensity, frequency, or type of exercises based on the patient's progress and feedback. If certain exercises are proving more beneficial or if new issues arise, therapists can adapt the program accordingly to address these changes. This dynamic approach ensures that therapy remains relevant and effective throughout the recovery process.

CHAPTER SIX

ALTERNATIVE AND COMPLEMENTARY THERAPIES

OVERVIEW OF POPULAR ALTERNATIVE TREATMENTS

Alternative treatments for Bell's Palsy often focus on enhancing overall well-being and supporting the body's natural healing processes. These treatments are sought by individuals looking for complementary methods to traditional medical care. Popular options include acupuncture, herbal remedies, and mind-body techniques such as meditation and yoga. These therapies aim to reduce symptoms and improve the quality of life by addressing both physical and emotional aspects of the condition. Each method brings unique approaches to managing Bell's Palsy, and understanding their distinct benefits can help in choosing the most suitable options.

Acupuncture, for instance, is a time-honored practice rooted in Traditional Chinese Medicine. It involves inserting fine needles into specific points on the body to balance energy flow and alleviate pain. This technique is believed to stimulate the nervous system and improve circulation, potentially aiding in nerve recovery and reducing inflammation associated with Bell's Palsy. Similarly, herbal remedies and supplements offer a range of natural compounds that may support nerve health and reduce inflammation, such as turmeric and ginger. These remedies are often used alongside conventional treatments to enhance therapeutic outcomes.

Mind-body techniques like meditation and yoga are integral to managing stress and promoting overall wellness, which can be beneficial for individuals with Bell's Palsy. Meditation helps to center the mind and reduce stress, which may contribute to better immune function and quicker recovery. Yoga, on the other hand, incorporates gentle stretching and breathing exercises that can improve facial muscle strength and flexibility, potentially aiding in symptom relief. By integrating these alternative therapies with traditional treatments, individuals may experience a more holistic approach to managing Bell's Palsy.

ACUPUNCTURE AND ITS BENEFITS

Acupuncture is an ancient practice that has been used for thousands of years to treat various conditions, including Bell's Palsy. The practice involves the insertion of very thin needles into specific acupuncture points on the body to restore balance and promote healing. For Bell's Palsy, acupuncture is thought to help by stimulating the nervous system, improving blood flow, and reducing inflammation around the affected facial nerves. This process may lead to improved facial muscle function and reduced symptoms.

Patients undergoing acupuncture for Bell's Palsy often report a reduction in pain and discomfort associated with the condition. Additionally, acupuncture sessions can help to relieve stress and anxiety, which are common for individuals dealing with the emotional and physical impacts of Bell's Palsy. By promoting relaxation and improving overall energy flow, acupuncture may contribute to a more balanced and effective recovery process. It's important to seek a qualified acupuncturist who is experienced in treating facial nerve conditions to ensure the best results.

Regular acupuncture treatments can complement conventional medical approaches, enhancing overall recovery and symptom management. Sessions are typically scheduled weekly, and the number of treatments required may vary depending on the individual's response and the severity of symptoms. By integrating acupuncture with other therapies, patients may benefit from a comprehensive approach to managing Bell's Palsy and improving their quality of life.

HERBAL REMEDIES AND SUPPLEMENTS

Herbal remedies and supplements offer a range of natural options for supporting nerve health and reducing inflammation in individuals with Bell's Palsy. Commonly used herbs include turmeric, known for its anti-inflammatory properties, and ginkgo biloba, which is believed to improve blood circulation and support nerve function. These natural remedies can be taken in various forms, such as capsules, teas, or tinctures, and are often used alongside conventional treatments to enhance overall effectiveness.

When incorporating herbal supplements into a treatment plan, it's crucial to consult with a healthcare provider to ensure that they do not interact with prescribed medications or existing health conditions. Dosages and potential side effects should be discussed to avoid adverse reactions.

Herbal remedies are typically considered safe when used as directed, but individual responses can vary, so monitoring for any changes in symptoms is important.

Supplementing with vitamins such as B-complex, particularly B12, may also support nerve health and aid in the recovery from Bell's Palsy.

These nutrients play a role in nerve repair and regeneration, and deficiencies can exacerbate symptoms. Combining herbal remedies with a balanced diet and regular medical care can provide a supportive and complementary approach to managing Bell's Palsy.

MIND-BODY TECHNIQUES (E.G., MEDITATION, YOGA)

Mind-body techniques, including meditation and yoga, are effective methods for managing the stress and physical symptoms associated with Bell's Palsy. Meditation involves practicing mindfulness and relaxation techniques to help calm the mind and reduce stress, which can be beneficial in alleviating the emotional impact of Bell's Palsy. By regularly engaging in meditation, individuals can improve their overall mental well-being and potentially aid in the body's healing processes.

Yoga is another valuable practice that incorporates physical movement, stretching, and deep breathing exercises.

For Bell's Palsy, gentle yoga poses can help to improve facial muscle strength and flexibility, which may assist in alleviating some of the physical symptoms. Additionally, yoga promotes relaxation and stress relief, which can be beneficial for individuals dealing with the emotional strain of the condition. Regular practice can enhance overall body awareness and support nerve recovery.

Both meditation and yoga can be easily incorporated into daily routines and offer a holistic approach to managing Bell's Palsy. By combining these techniques with other treatments, individuals may experience a more balanced approach to their recovery, addressing both the physical and emotional aspects of the condition. Beginners can start with short sessions and gradually increase the duration as they become more comfortable with the practices.

EVALUATING EFFECTIVENESS AND SAFETY

When exploring alternative therapies for Bell's Palsy, evaluating their effectiveness and safety is essential to ensure they contribute positively to the recovery process. This involves assessing how well the treatments work in alleviating symptoms and improving overall quality of life. Research and clinical studies can provide valuable insights into the efficacy of various alternative therapies, such as acupuncture, herbal remedies, and mind-body techniques.

Safety considerations are equally important, as some alternative treatments may interact with conventional medications or have potential side effects. Consulting with healthcare professionals before starting any new therapy is crucial to avoid complications and ensure that the chosen treatments are appropriate for the individual's specific condition. Tracking any changes in symptoms and discussing them with a healthcare provider can help in adjusting the treatment plan as needed.

A well-rounded approach to evaluating alternative therapies includes not only considering scientific evidence but also personal experiences and preferences.

CHAPTER SEVEN

MANAGING COMPLICATIONS

COMMON COMPLICATIONS AND THEIR SYMPTOMS

Bell's Palsy, a condition affecting the facial nerves, can lead to a range of complications, each presenting with distinct symptoms. Common complications include persistent facial weakness, where one side of the face may remain less expressive than the other and involuntary facial twitching or spasms, which can be unsettling. Additionally, some individuals experience dry eyes or excessive tearing due to disrupted control over the tear glands. These symptoms can affect daily activities and overall comfort.

Another notable complication is difficulty in closing the eye on the affected side, which can lead to dryness or irritation. This often results from impaired control over the muscles responsible for blinking. Patients may also encounter challenges with eating and speaking, as facial muscle weakness can affect lip control and expression. Recognizing these symptoms early is crucial for effective management and treatment.

Lastly, Bell's Palsy can cause altered taste sensation on the front two-thirds of the tongue. This can affect appetite and enjoyment of food. Sensory disturbances may also occur, including numbness or tingling in the affected area. Identifying these symptoms can help differentiate Bell's Palsy from other conditions and guide appropriate treatment measures.

STRATEGIES TO MANAGE FACIAL PAIN AND DISCOMFORT

Managing facial pain and discomfort associated with Bell's Palsy involves several practical strategies. Applying warm or cold compresses to the affected area can help alleviate pain and reduce inflammation. Alternating between heat and cold packs may provide relief from discomfort and help soothe irritated nerves. It is essential to use a comfortable temperature to avoid skin damage.

Over-the-counter pain medications, such as acetaminophen or ibuprofen, can be effective in managing mild to moderate pain. These medications help reduce inflammation and provide relief from discomfort. It's important to follow dosing instructions and consult with a healthcare provider if pain persists or worsens, as they can offer guidance on more potent pain relief options.

Gentle facial exercises and massage can also aid in reducing discomfort and improving muscle function.

Massaging the affected side of the face with a light touch can stimulate blood flow and alleviate tension.

ADDRESSING ISSUES WITH FACIAL WEAKNESS

Facial weakness resulting from Bell's Palsy requires targeted strategies to address and manage the condition effectively. Performing facial exercises, as recommended by a healthcare provider, can help strengthen weakened muscles and improve facial symmetry. These exercises might include raising the eyebrows, closing the eyes tightly, and smiling. Consistent practice of these exercises can promote muscle recovery and function.

Using adaptive techniques for daily activities can also support individuals coping with facial weakness. For instance, utilizing straw or special utensils can assist with eating and drinking, making it easier to manage. Speech therapy may also be beneficial in addressing communication challenges related to facial weakness, helping individuals articulate more clearly and effectively.

Incorporating facial muscle stimulation techniques, such as electrical stimulation therapy, may be recommended by a healthcare professional. This therapy involves applying gentle electrical currents to the facial muscles to enhance their strength and coordination. This approach, when used in conjunction with exercises and adaptive techniques, can support the recovery process and improve facial function.

COPING WITH EMOTIONAL AND PSYCHOLOGICAL CHALLENGES

Dealing with the emotional and psychological impact of Bell's Palsy is a significant aspect of managing the condition. The sudden onset of facial weakness can affect self-esteem and body image, leading to feelings of frustration or sadness.

Seeking support from mental health professionals or support groups can be invaluable in addressing these emotional challenges. Sharing experiences and receiving guidance from others facing similar issues can provide comfort and coping strategies.

Developing a positive mindset and focusing on recovery goals can help manage the psychological impact of Bell's Palsy. Setting small, achievable goals and celebrating progress, no matter how minor, can foster a sense of accomplishment and motivation.

Engaging in activities that boost self-esteem and relaxation, such as hobbies or mindfulness practices, can also aid in emotional well-being.

Additionally, educating oneself about Bell's Palsy and its potential outcomes can alleviate anxiety and uncertainty. Understanding that the condition often improves over time and that various treatment options are available can provide reassurance. Staying informed and actively participating in one's treatment plan can empower individuals to face the challenges of Bell's Palsy with greater confidence.

SEEKING ADDITIONAL MEDICAL SUPPORT

When Bell's Palsy symptoms persist or complications arise, seeking additional medical support is essential. Consulting with a neurologist or a specialist in facial disorders can provide a comprehensive evaluation and advanced treatment options. These specialists can offer tailored advice on managing symptoms, exploring new therapies, and monitoring progress.

In some cases, physical therapy or rehabilitation services may be recommended to support muscle recovery and function. Physical therapists can design personalized exercise programs and provide hands-on treatments to enhance facial strength and coordination. Regular follow-up appointments with healthcare providers can help track progress and make necessary adjustments to the treatment plan.

Exploring complementary therapies, such as acupuncture or biofeedback, may also be beneficial for managing symptoms and promoting overall well-being. These alternative approaches can offer additional support alongside conventional treatments, providing a holistic approach to managing Bell's Palsy. It is important to discuss any new therapies with healthcare providers to ensure they are appropriate and safe.

CHAPTER EIGHT

LONG-TERM OUTLOOK AND PROGNOSIS

EXPECTED RECOVERY RATES

Bell's palsy often presents an unpredictable journey, but many individuals experience significant improvement within three to six months. The majority of patients recover fully or nearly fully, with around 70% regaining normal facial function. Recovery rates can vary based on the severity of the initial symptoms and the speed of treatment. Early intervention with medications like corticosteroids can enhance recovery chances and reduce the risk of long-term complications.

For some, recovery may be slower, extending beyond six months. These individuals might experience residual weakness or asymmetry in the facial muscles. The extent of recovery can be influenced by factors such as age, overall health, and the presence of other medical conditions.

Regular assessment by healthcare professionals can provide insights into the expected recovery timeline and necessary interventions.

It's crucial to manage expectations and understand that while many people achieve full recovery, others may have varying degrees of residual symptoms. Continuing medical advice and adhering to prescribed treatments can support optimal recovery outcomes and help in adjusting expectations based on individual progress.

LONG-TERM EFFECTS AND POTENTIAL RESIDUAL SYMPTOMS

Even with treatment, some individuals with Bell's palsy may encounter long-term effects or residual symptoms. These can include facial weakness, involuntary movements, or difficulty with facial expressions. In some cases, the affected side of the face might exhibit persistent muscle tone imbalances, leading to subtle asymmetries or functional challenges.

Dry eye, changes in taste, and sensitivity to sound on the affected side are other potential long-term effects. These residual symptoms can impact daily life and emotional well-being, making it essential to address them proactively. Symptom management strategies such as physical therapy, facial exercises, and lubrication for the eyes can help alleviate discomfort and improve quality of life.

Understanding that these residual effects are possible helps in preparing for ongoing care and adjustments in daily routines. Collaborating with healthcare providers to develop a tailored management plan can assist in addressing and minimizing the impact of any lasting symptoms.

FACTORS AFFECTING LONG-TERM PROGNOSIS

Several factors can influence the long-term prognosis of Bell's palsy. Early diagnosis and prompt initiation of treatment are crucial in improving outcomes. The severity of the initial symptoms plays a significant role; more severe cases may have a higher likelihood of residual effects. Additionally, the patient's age, general health, and presence of comorbid conditions can affect recovery rates and the extent of symptom resolution.

Genetic predispositions and underlying autoimmune conditions can also impact long-term recovery. Research suggests that individuals with pre-existing health issues or those who experience severe initial symptoms might face more challenges in achieving complete recovery. Tailoring treatment plans to these individual factors can aid in better management and improved long-term outcomes.

Ongoing evaluation by medical professionals helps in assessing how these factors interplay in each case.

IMPORTANCE OF ONGOING MEDICAL FOLLOW-UP

Ongoing medical follow-up is essential for managing Bell's palsy and optimizing recovery. Regular check-ups with a healthcare provider help monitor progress, address complications, and adjust treatment plans as needed. Follow-up visits can include assessments of facial function, evaluation of any residual symptoms, and adjustments to medications or therapies.

Consistent follow-up allows for early identification of any new or worsening symptoms, enabling timely intervention. It also provides an opportunity for healthcare providers to offer support, answer questions, and guide patients through the recovery process. This ongoing relationship helps ensure that patients receive the most effective care and support tailored to their evolving needs.

Maintaining a regular schedule of medical appointments and staying engaged with the treatment plan is critical for achieving the best possible outcomes.

SUPPORT NETWORKS AND RESOURCES

Support networks and resources play a vital role in managing Bell's palsy and enhancing recovery.

Engaging with support groups, both online and in-person, can provide emotional support and practical advice from others who have experienced similar challenges. These networks offer a platform for sharing experiences, coping strategies, and encouragement, which can be beneficial for emotional well-being.

Access to resources such as physical therapy, speech therapy, and counseling can aid in addressing specific symptoms and improving overall function. Many communities offer specialized services and programs designed to support individuals with Bell's palsy, including educational workshops and rehabilitative therapies.

Connecting with healthcare professionals, support groups, and community resources provides a comprehensive approach to managing Bell's palsy. Leveraging these networks helps individuals navigate their recovery journey with enhanced support and access to valuable information and services.

CHAPTER NINE

LIVING WITH BELL'S PALSY

ADJUSTING TO DAILY LIFE WITH BELL'S PALSY

Living with Bell's Palsy can bring significant changes to daily routines due to facial weakness or paralysis. It's essential to adapt your home environment to accommodate these changes. Simple adjustments, such as using hands-free devices for phone calls or installing grab bars in the bathroom, can make daily activities easier and safer. Meals might need to be modified to accommodate difficulties with chewing or swallowing, and using softer foods can alleviate discomfort.

Personal grooming routines may also need to be adapted. Using tools like electric razors for shaving or specialized toothbrushes can help manage the challenges of facial weakness. If facial expressions are affected, it's useful to practice facial exercises recommended by healthcare providers to maintain muscle tone and improve control over facial movements.

Finally, keeping a consistent routine can help manage the unpredictability of Bell's Palsy. Establishing a structured schedule for tasks such as taking medications, attending therapy sessions, and engaging in physical exercises can help maintain a sense of normalcy and control. Support from family members in managing these routines can also be beneficial in easing the adjustment process.

COPING STRATEGIES AND SUPPORT SYSTEMS

Coping with Bell's Palsy often involves finding effective strategies to manage the emotional and physical aspects of the condition.

Developing a coping strategy that includes relaxation techniques, such as deep breathing or meditation, can help reduce stress and anxiety associated with the condition. Learning to recognize and address stress triggers can be crucial in maintaining overall well-being.

Support systems play a vital role in coping with Bell's Palsy. Engaging with family, friends, or support groups can provide emotional encouragement and practical advice. It's also helpful to connect with healthcare professionals who can offer tailored guidance and recommend effective treatments or therapies to manage symptoms and improve quality of life.

Additionally, setting realistic goals and celebrating small victories can enhance coping strategies. Focusing on gradual improvements and acknowledging progress can boost morale and motivate to continue with treatment and rehabilitation efforts.

MANAGING SOCIAL AND WORK-RELATED CHALLENGES

Navigating social interactions and work-related activities can be particularly challenging for those with Bell's Palsy. At work, it might be necessary to discuss accommodations with your employer, such as flexible work hours or tasks that minimize physical strain. Being open about your condition with colleagues can also help create a supportive work environment.

Socially, managing Bell's Palsy requires patience and understanding from friends and family. It can be helpful to educate them about the condition to foster empathy and reduce any misunderstandings. Engaging in social activities that are comfortable and enjoyable can also help maintain social connections and improve self-esteem.

Adapting communication methods might be necessary for social interactions. Using written communication or technology-assisted methods can assist in conveying messages when facial expressions are impaired. Finding alternative ways to engage in social and professional settings can help maintain a sense of normalcy and participation.

IMPORTANCE OF MENTAL HEALTH AND WELL-BEING

Maintaining mental health and well-being is crucial for individuals with Bell's Palsy. The emotional impact of facing physical changes can be significant, so prioritizing mental health through therapy or counseling can provide valuable support. Mental health professionals can offer strategies for coping with emotional challenges and building resilience.

Engaging in activities that promote mental well-being, such as hobbies or exercise, can also be beneficial. These activities can serve as distractions from the condition and contribute to a more positive outlook. Regular physical activity, when suitable, can help reduce symptoms of anxiety and depression.

Building a strong support network is essential for mental health. Connecting with others who understand the challenges of Bell's Palsy can provide a sense of community and shared experience.

ENGAGING WITH PATIENT COMMUNITIES AND SUPPORT GROUPS

Connecting with patient communities and support groups can provide valuable resources and emotional support for those with Bell's Palsy. These groups offer opportunities to share experiences, exchange advice, and learn from others facing similar challenges. Participating in discussions and events can also foster a sense of belonging and reduce feelings of isolation.

Support groups often provide practical tips and information about managing symptoms and accessing treatments. They may host educational sessions or workshops that can help individuals stay informed about the latest research and therapies available for Bell's Palsy.

Additionally, engaging with patient communities can be empowering. By sharing personal stories and supporting others, individuals with Bell's Palsy can contribute to a collective understanding and help advocate for better resources and awareness.

CHAPTER TEN

COMMON CONCERNS AND DETAILED FAQS

WHAT ARE THE EARLY SIGNS OF BELL'S PALSY?

Bell's Palsy often begins with a sudden weakness or paralysis on one side of the face, which may develop rapidly within hours. Individuals might notice that one side of their face droops, making it difficult to close one eye, smile, or raise their eyebrows. This asymmetry is typically noticeable when trying to perform facial expressions.

Additional early signs include a tingling or numb sensation in the affected area, which can sometimes be accompanied by pain around the jaw or behind the ear.

Some people experience an increased sensitivity to sound on the affected side, and changes in taste on the front part of the tongue may also occur. These symptoms often appear without warning and can be distressing.

It's important to seek medical attention if these symptoms arise, as early diagnosis and treatment can improve outcomes. Doctors often conduct a physical examination and may use imaging tests to differentiate Bell's Palsy from other conditions.

HOW IS BELL'S PALSY DIFFERENTIATED FROM A STROKE?

Bell's Palsy and strokes can present with facial weakness, but they have distinct differences. In Bell's Palsy, facial weakness is usually isolated to one side of the face and affects the entire side, including the forehead, which distinguishes it from strokes. Stroke-related facial weakness often spares the forehead, leaving the brow unaffected.

A stroke might present with additional symptoms such as sudden confusion, difficulty speaking, or loss of balance, which are not typical of Bell's Palsy. Medical professionals use a combination of physical examination and imaging studies, such as CT scans or MRIs, to determine the underlying cause of facial weakness.

Rapid differentiation is crucial because the treatments for Bell's Palsy and strokes differ significantly. While Bell's Palsy is often treated with medications and physical therapy, strokes require emergency interventions to address the underlying cause and prevent further damage.

WHAT ARE THE MOST EFFECTIVE TREATMENTS AVAILABLE?

The primary treatment for Bell's Palsy often includes corticosteroids, such as prednisone, to reduce inflammation and swelling of the facial nerve. Early administration of these medications is crucial for reducing the severity and duration of symptoms. Pain relievers and antiviral medications may also be prescribed if a viral infection is suspected to be a contributing factor.

Physical therapy plays a significant role in recovery by helping to maintain muscle tone and prevent stiffness in the facial muscles. Facial exercises can aid in improving facial symmetry and functionality. Additionally, using warm compresses can alleviate pain and discomfort associated with Bell's Palsy.

In some cases, if symptoms persist beyond a few months, alternative treatments such as acupuncture or surgical options might be considered. Regular follow-ups with a healthcare provider are essential to monitor progress and adjust treatments as needed.

CAN BELL'S PALSY RECUR OR AFFECT BOTH SIDES OF THE FACE?

Bell's Palsy typically affects one side of the face, but recurrence is possible. While rare, some individuals may experience Bell's Palsy more than once, though it usually remains unilateral. Each episode can vary in severity and duration, with many people recovering fully after a single occurrence.

In very rare cases, Bell's Palsy can affect both sides of the face, a condition known as bilateral Bell's Palsy.

This is less common and often requires further investigation to rule out other medical conditions or underlying issues that could be contributing to the bilateral symptoms.

Monitoring for any new or recurring symptoms is important, as early intervention can help manage the condition effectively. Consulting with a healthcare provider can guide preventive measures and address any concerns regarding recurrence.

HOW CAN I FIND SUPPORT AND RESOURCES FOR BELL'S PALSY?

Finding support for Bell's Palsy involves accessing a range of resources, including healthcare providers, support groups, and online communities. Many organizations offer information on treatment options, coping strategies, and ongoing research about Bell's Palsy.

Support groups, both online and in-person, can provide emotional support and practical advice from individuals who have experienced similar challenges. These groups often share personal experiences, recovery tips, and recommendations for managing daily life with Bell's Palsy.

Local and national organizations dedicated to neurological disorders can offer additional resources, including educational materials, advocacy, and financial assistance for treatment. Connecting with these resources can provide valuable support and help individuals navigate their journey with Bell's Palsy.

www.ingramcontent.com/pod-product-compliance
Lightning Source LLC
Chambersburg PA
CBHW061300250726
48653CB00002B/709